FAMILY CARE

NAVIGATING ELDER CARE WITH COMPASSION AND WISDOM

B. MARWO

Disclaimer

The information provided in this book is intended for educational and informational purposes only. It is based on personal experiences and research and should not be construed as professional medical advice. The author, B. Marwo, is not a licensed healthcare provider and this book should not replace consultations with qualified professionals in the field.

Readers are encouraged to consult with appropriate professionals before making decisions regarding elder care. The author disclaims any liability for any direct or indirect consequences resulting from the use or application of the information contained in this book.

Every effort has been made to ensure the accuracy of the content at the time of publication. However, the author does not assume responsibility for errors, omissions, or changes that may occur after the publication date.

Family Care: Navigating Elder Care with Compassion and Wisdom

B. MARWO

TABLE OF CONTENTS

Caring for an elderly family member is a deeply personal journey. It comes with its emotional highs and physical challenges, especially when health issues or mobility limitations come into play. The key to being an effective caregiver is understanding the unique needs of the elderly—whether they're dealing with memory loss, physical disabilities, or simply navigating the aging process. Having this insight will not only make your role easier but will also ensure they feel cared for with dignity and respect.

Physical Needs: Mobility and Hygiene

One of the first challenges you'll face is assisting with mobility. When my aunt began to lose her balance and strength, we quickly realized that even simple tasks—like getting in and out of bed— required careful attention. For those dealing with severe physical limitations, such as arthritis or stroke, mobility becomes even more complex.

Women, in particular, need extra care when it comes to hygiene. When my aunt became bedridden, we had to be especially mindful of infections like yeast infections, which are more common when hygiene is compromised. I learned that using gentle, unscented products and frequently changing incontinence products made a significant difference. These small acts of care preserved her comfort and dignity, even during her most vulnerable moments.

Assistive devices like walkers, grab bars, or even wheelchairs can help ease their day-to-day life. Encourage small movements throughout the day to maintain muscle strength and circulation. Even when movement is limited, stretching or shifting weight can reduce stiffness and prevent pressure sores, a common issue for those who are less mobile. Have you ever noticed how a simple walk around the garden or a few minutes of light stretching can brighten someone's day?

Cognitive Needs: Patience and Connection

Memory loss is perhaps one of the most challenging aspects of elderly care. My neighbor told me about the first time her husband forgot her birthday. At first, it stung, but she soon realized it wasn't his fault—it was the result of age. Whether your loved one is dealing with mild forgetfulness or more severe conditions like dementia or Alzheimer's, patience is your greatest tool.

It can be frustrating to repeat yourself or answer the same question multiple times, but remember, they aren't doing it on purpose. Instead of showing irritation, try redirecting the conversation. If your loved one keeps asking about long-gone appointments or events, gently steer them toward something positive: "Why don't we look through the photo album instead?"

Reading together can also help strengthen the bond between you and your elderly loved one. When my aunt's memory started to fade, I began reading to her from her bible. She couldn't always follow the story, but it brought her comfort to hear the familiar words. How many of us take the time to simply sit and read aloud to those we care for? These small moments of connection can be deeply healing.

Emotional Needs: Involvement and Autonomy

As physical and cognitive abilities decline, many elderly individuals feel like they're losing control of their lives. My uncle once confided, "It's like the world keeps moving while I'm stuck in place." That sense of being left behind is common, but it can be alleviated by involving them in decisions—no matter how small.

Whether it's choosing their clothes for the day or deciding on a meal, including them in these choices helps maintain their autonomy. Have you ever thought about how empowering it can be for someone to simply choose what they'll have for dinner? These decisions, small as they may seem, can preserve their dignity and independence. My aunt, even as her health declined, always loved picking out which flowers to plant in the garden, and it gave her a sense of ownership over her space.

Elderly individuals also need strong advocates—especially in medical settings where their voices can easily be drowned out. When my uncle was hospitalized, I became his spokesperson, making sure the doctors explained every decision in terms he could understand. It's important to ensure that they remain at the center of their own care decisions.

Nutrition and Hydration

As people age, their nutritional needs change. You might notice that your loved one eats less, or has difficulty chewing. My grand-aunt struggled with this after a stroke left her with reduced appetite and difficulty swallowing. Ensuring she got enough nutrients became a priority.

Elderly individuals often require fewer calories, but their need for vitamins and minerals remains high. Their meals should be rich in protein, fiber, and essential nutrients to maintain strength and support overall health. I found that offering small, nutrient-dense meals more frequently throughout the day worked better than expecting my grand-aunt to eat large portions.

Protein is especially important in preventing muscle loss, which is a common issue with aging. Foods like eggs, fish, and soft-cooked chicken have to be staples in the household. For those who struggle with chewing or swallowing, smoothies, mashed vegetables, and yogurt can be easier to manage while still providing necessary nutrients. Wouldn't you agree that even simple meals can be powerful when prepared thoughtfully?

Hydration is equally important, yet many elderly people don't drink enough water. Dehydration can lead to confusion, urinary tract infections, and other complications. My uncle often forgets to drink, so we place water bottles in his favorite spots— by the TV, on the table near his chair. Have you ever thought about how easy it is to overlook such a simple need?

Encourage fluids throughout the day—water, herbal teas, and water-rich foods like cucumbers or watermelon are great options. If your loved one resists plain water, try adding a slice of lemon or cucumber for flavor. This small adjustment can make all the difference in keeping them hydrated and healthy.

Practical Tips for Understanding Needs:

- Conduct daily check-ins to assess both physical and emotional well-being.

- Develop a routine for mobility and hygiene care, especially for those with severe disabilities

- Use memory aids or photo albums to stimulate memory in gentle ways.

- Always include them in decisions that affect their daily life, no matter how small.

In understanding their needs holistically—physical, cognitive, and emotional—you'll create a caregiving environment filled with compassion and respect. Every challenge becomes easier to navigate with empathy, and your loved one will feel more valued and secure. After all, isn't that the heart of caregiving?

Mobility is one of the most important aspects of an elderly person's independence. As people age, mobility often becomes limited due to factors like arthritis, muscle weakness, balance issues, or medical conditions. Ensuring that your loved one remains as mobile as possible is key to maintaining their sense of independence and preventing injuries. In this episode, we'll cover practical tips for assisting with mobility and ensuring their physical safety while respecting their dignity.

Assessing Their Mobility Needs

The first step in supporting your loved one's mobility is to assess their current level of independence. Do they need help standing up or sitting down? Are they unsteady on their feet? Do they use a cane or walker? A physical therapist or doctor can help you determine what level of support they need and provide guidance on the right mobility aids.

Mobility aids like canes, walkers, or wheelchairs are invaluable tools that can help maintain independence. However, it's important to choose the right tool for their abilities and ensure they are using it correctly. Sometimes, resistance to these aids arises from fear of losing independence, but framing these tools as a way to stay active and safe rather than as a sign of decline can make them more acceptable.

Preventing Falls and Injuries

Falls are one of the leading causes of injury in the elderly, and preventing them is a top priority. Small adjustments in their living space can greatly reduce the risk of falls. Start by ensuring that their home is free of clutter and that walkways are clear. Remove loose rugs or secure them with non-slip backing, and make sure that any spills are cleaned up immediately to prevent slipping.

Consider installing handrails in hallways, bathrooms, and along stairs. Grab bars near the toilet and in the shower can provide additional support where it's most needed. Proper lighting is also essential—make sure rooms and hallways are well-lit, and add nightlights to areas they may walk through in the dark, such as the path to the bathroom.

Encourage your loved one to wear supportive, non-slip shoes rather than slippers or socks that can increase the risk of slipping. If they have trouble seeing, consider getting their vision checked regularly to ensure they aren't at additional risk due to poor eyesight.

Assisting with Mobility

When helping your loved one move from one place to another, it's important to do so in a way that preserves their dignity while ensuring their safety. Offer your arm for support or gently guide them from behind, but allow them to move as independently as possible. It can be tempting to take over and do everything for them, but allowing them to move on their own is crucial for maintaining their physical strength and confidence.

If they use a wheelchair, make sure they are comfortable and positioned correctly. Always lock the wheelchair when they are getting in or out, and help them transfer safely by guiding their movements rather than lifting them entirely, if possible. Using a gait belt can provide extra stability when transferring between surfaces.

Exercises for Strength and Balance

Keeping your loved one active is key to maintaining their mobility and preventing further decline. Even if they have limited mobility, there are exercises they can do to strengthen their muscles and improve balance. Seated exercises, leg lifts, or gentle stretching can help improve flexibility and reduce stiffness. For those who are more mobile, walking, swimming, or using resistance bands can maintain strength and endurance.

Encourage your loved one to stay active in ways that are enjoyable to them. Going for short walks in the garden or dancing to their favorite music can be both fun and beneficial for their physical health. Even if they are mostly chair-bound, engaging in arm exercises or light stretching can boost circulation and help maintain flexibility.

Encouraging Independence

As much as possible, allow your loved one to move independently. This may mean letting them take extra time to complete tasks or walk at their own pace. Patience is key. It's important to strike a balance between keeping them safe and not overprotecting them to the point where they lose confidence in their abilities.

Encourage them to do activities they enjoy that also promote mobility. Gardening, cooking, or light housework can all be modified to suit their abilities while keeping them active. Having them involved in these daily tasks not only maintains their physical strength but also supports their emotional well-being by giving them a sense of purpose and autonomy.

Safety Equipment

In addition to mobility aids, consider safety equipment that can assist with mobility in and around the home. Raised toilet seats, shower chairs, and bed rails can make everyday tasks easier and safer. If they struggle with balance, using a transfer bench to help them get in and out of the shower can prevent slips.

If your loved one is at high risk of falling, a medical alert system can provide an added layer of security. These devices allow them to call for help at the push of a button if they fall or have an emergency while alone. Knowing they have this option can ease both your concerns and theirs.

Practical Tips for Supporting Mobility:

- Assess their mobility needs and consult with a professional for appropriate aids like walkers or canes.

- Remove fall hazards from their home and install safety features like handrails and grab bars.

- Assist with mobility in a way that promotes their independence and dignity.

- Encourage strength-building exercises, no matter their mobility level.

- Incorporate fun, active tasks into their daily routine to keep them engaged and mobile.

Maintaining mobility is key to your loved one's sense of independence and overall health. By providing the right support, you can help them stay safe and active for as long as possible. In the next episode, we'll dive into personal hygiene and how to handle these sensitive tasks with dignity and care.

Communication is at the heart of caregiving. Whether your elderly loved one is experiencing memory loss, hearing difficulties, or simply the frustration that comes with aging, the way you communicate with them can either build a bridge or a wall. Good communication fosters trust and reduces misunderstandings, while poor communication can lead to frustration, confusion, or even resentment.

Speak Clearly and Gently

As seniors age, hearing can become less sharp, which often leads to misunderstandings. It's crucial to speak clearly and at a moderate pace. You don't need to shout but ensure your tone is calm and your words are enunciated. Eye contact is key—it helps them focus and makes it easier for them to read your facial expressions, which can be helpful when words are hard to hear or process.

One thing to avoid is "talking down" to them, which can make them feel infantilized. Even if their cognitive abilities have declined, they still deserve the respect that clear, straightforward communication brings. Use simple language if needed, but speak as you would to anyone else—with patience and kindness.

Be Their Voice and Advocate

As your loved one ages, they might feel powerless in many situations, especially when it comes to healthcare. Being their voice is critical. This means not only speaking up for them in medical settings but also ensuring they understand what's happening. Doctors often use medical jargon that can confuse patients, so be sure to explain things in simpler terms afterward, if necessary.

It's equally important to let your elderly loved one express their concerns. Even if they struggle with memory or decision-making, their input matters. They might fear their wishes being overridden by doctors or other family members. You can help by asking them open-ended questions like, "How do you feel about this medication?" or "Do you want to ask the doctor something?" This shows them that they are not being sidelined, and their voice still counts.

Managing Memory Loss: Patience Is Key

If your elderly loved one is dealing with memory loss or dementia, communication can become even more challenging. Repetition is often needed, and it can test your patience. Instead of becoming frustrated when they forget something you've said multiple times, try to see things from their perspective. They aren't forgetting on purpose—it's a symptom of their condition.

Gentle reminders or visual aids can be helpful. Use notes, pictures, or daily schedules to orient them. For example, if they frequently ask what day it is, having a large calendar in a visible place can help reduce confusion. Keeping instructions simple and breaking them down into smaller steps can also make it easier for them to follow along.

Involvement in Decision-Making

No matter how much cognitive decline they may face, seniors deserve to be included in decisions. Whether it's as small as what they want to eat for lunch or as big as discussing healthcare plans, their opinions should be sought. Involving them in decisions shows them that they still have autonomy and that their preferences matter.

For example, you can ask, "Would you prefer to go for a walk today or read a book together?" or "Do you want to wear the blue sweater or the red one?" These choices might seem trivial, but they provide your elderly loved one with a sense of control over their life, which can improve their mental well-being.

Active Listening: More Than Just Words

When communicating with seniors, listening is just as important as speaking. Active listening involves more than just hearing their words—it's about understanding their emotions, even if they struggle to articulate them. Pay attention to body language, facial expressions, and tone. Sometimes a simple "How are you feeling today?" can open the door to deeper conversations about fears, frustrations, or needs they may not express outright.

By being attentive, you'll build a sense of trust, and they'll feel more comfortable sharing their thoughts and feelings with you. This is especially important if they're reluctant to discuss difficult subjects like pain, discomfort, or sadness.

Practical Communication Tips:

- Always face them when speaking and make eye contact.

- Use simple words but avoid speaking down to them.

- Be patient when they forget things and use gentle reminders.

- Include them in decision-making, no matter how small the decision.

- Actively listen—pay attention to both what they say and how they say it.

Good communication can transform your caregiving experience. By speaking clearly, listening actively, and showing patience, you'll foster a stronger connection with your loved one, helping them feel respected and valued. Next, we'll dive into the hands-on aspects of providing physical care, from hygiene to mobility assistance

Personal hygiene is an intimate and often sensitive area when caring for the elderly. As they age, your loved one may face challenges that make maintaining hygiene difficult, whether due to mobility issues, illness, or cognitive decline. Assisting them in this area is crucial for their health and well-being, but it must be handled with respect to preserve their dignity. In this chapter, we'll explore strategies for providing personal care with compassion and maintaining their hygiene without compromising their self-esteem.

Understanding the Importance of Hygiene

Good personal hygiene is not just about cleanliness; it is also key to preventing infections and other health issues. As we age, the skin becomes more delicate and susceptible to infections such as bed sores, especially for those who are less mobile or bedridden. Proper hygiene, from regular bathing to oral care, can prevent these issues and keep your loved one feeling fresh and comfortable.

In addition to physical health, hygiene plays a significant role in emotional well-being. Neglecting personal care can lead to feelings of embarrassment, low self-worth, and depression. When you step in to help, remember that you're not just addressing a physical need, but also helping them maintain their dignity.

Bathing and Grooming

Bathing can be one of the most difficult aspects of caregiving, especially if your loved one resists help or is embarrassed by their inability to manage this basic task. To make the process easier for both of you, establish a routine that feels natural and non-intrusive. Approach the task with kindness, explaining what you are doing at each step to put them at ease. If possible, allow them to do as much as they can on their own. Set them up with the tools they need—like a long-handled sponge or shower chair—so they can maintain some independence during bath time. For those with mobility challenges, sponge baths are a good alternative, ensuring they still get clean without the risk of falling in the shower or tub.

When assisting with grooming, such as brushing hair or shaving, be gentle and respectful. These tasks can help them feel like themselves again. Ask their preference for things like hairstyles, shaving routines, or which lotions they like to use. A warm towel, familiar scents, and gentle care can transform hygiene into a comforting experience.

Managing Incontinence

Incontinence is a sensitive topic that many elderly people find difficult to discuss. It can be an uncomfortable issue, both physically and emotionally, but it's important to approach it without judgment. Let your loved one know that this is a common part of aging and that there's nothing to be ashamed of.

There are several practical ways to manage incontinence, such as using protective undergarments, ensuring regular bathroom breaks, and providing easy access to the bathroom. For those who are bedridden, using absorbent pads or adult diapers can help keep them dry and prevent skin irritation. Always check and change these products frequently to prevent discomfort or infections.

Maintaining proper hygiene is crucial for those dealing with incontinence. Help them stay clean by gently washing the affected areas and applying barrier creams to protect the skin. Respect their privacy as much as possible, and reassure them that their comfort and dignity are your priority.

Feminine Hygiene

Women, in particular, face additional challenges as they age, including the need for extra attention to feminine hygiene. Urinary tract infections and other issues can arise if proper care is not taken. To prevent these problems, make sure your loved one changes their undergarments regularly and stays clean and dry, especially after using the restroom.

When assisting with feminine hygiene, handle the situation with utmost sensitivity. It can feel invasive, so it's important to maintain a calm, gentle demeanor and give them as much control over the process as possible. Be mindful of their comfort and preferences, and involve them in decisions about products like wipes, powders, or creams.

If they are prone to infections, consider consulting with their healthcare provider for advice on specific products or routines that can help prevent recurring issues. Keeping lines of communication open will ensure they feel comfortable discussing any concerns they have.

Dental Care

Oral hygiene is often overlooked in elderly care but is essential for overall health. Poor dental care can lead to painful conditions like gum disease or infections, which can affect their ability to eat properly and even lead to more serious health issues.

If your loved one is able, encourage them to brush their teeth at least twice a day and floss regularly. For those with limited mobility or cognitive decline, assist them by gently guiding their hand or using a toothbrush with a larger handle for better grip. If they wear dentures, ensure that they are cleaned daily and removed overnight to prevent infections or sores.

Regular dental checkups are also important. If your loved one finds it difficult to visit a dentist, many practices offer mobile services or in-home visits. Maintaining oral hygiene can go a long way in promoting their comfort and health.

Respecting Their Dignity

One of the most important things to remember when assisting with personal hygiene is to respect your loved one's dignity. Even if they need help with intimate tasks, they are still adults and deserve to be treated with respect and care. Always involve them in the process, asking for their preferences and allowing them to take the lead wherever possible.

Offer privacy by closing the door or stepping out of the room when appropriate. Speak calmly and with reassurance, and never rush through the process. Acknowledging their feelings, offering choices, and maintaining a gentle touch can make a world of difference in how they experience hygiene care.

Practical Tips for Maintaining Hygiene:

- Establish a regular hygiene routine that respects their dignity and independence.

- Assist with bathing, grooming, and dental care, allowing them to participate as much as possible.

- Manage incontinence with practical solutions like protective garments and frequent bathroom breaks.

- Pay special attention to feminine hygiene to prevent infections.

- Respect their need for privacy and make hygiene care a positive, comfortable experience.

Personal hygiene is an essential part of caregiving, and by handling it with compassion and respect, you can help your loved one maintain their health, comfort, and dignity.

When caring for an elderly loved one, many of the challenges center around providing hands-on physical care. From assisting with mobility to managing hygiene, creating a consistent routine can ease both your workload and their comfort. However, physical care requires sensitivity, as your loved one may feel vulnerable or embarrassed when others help with tasks they once did independently. The key is to approach each aspect of their care with compassion and respect.

Assisting with Mobility

One of the biggest challenges for caregivers is helping elderly individuals with limited mobility. Whether due to conditions like arthritis, stroke, or amputations, movement often becomes painful or difficult. If your loved one has had an amputation, the challenges are even more significant, requiring careful attention to their comfort and health.

Limited movement increases the risk of bed sores, which can lead to serious infections. You can prevent this by ensuring regular position changes and using special cushioning to relieve pressure on vulnerable areas like the back, elbows, and hips. Check for redness or irritation daily, as early detection is key to preventing skin breakdown

For those who are less mobile, pressure sores (commonly called bed sores) are a major risk. These sores develop when the skin breaks down due to prolonged pressure on one area. To prevent this, make sure your loved one changes positions regularly, at least every two hours. You can use pillows to help prop them up in a new position, ensuring that pressure is distributed evenly.

Regular movement—whether it's a gentle walk or simply moving from a chair to the bed—helps maintain muscle tone and circulation. If mobility is extremely limited, even small movements, like shifting weight or rotating their arms and legs, can make a difference.

Maintaining Proper Hygiene

Hygiene is an essential part of daily care, and it's important for both physical health and dignity. Many elderly individuals may be unable to bathe or perform personal care independently, which can be a sensitive issue. Approach these tasks with care, making sure they feel comfortable and respected.

For bedridden or less mobile women, it's crucial to maintain cleanliness in intimate areas by using gentle, unscented products and changing incontinence pads or garments frequently. This not only preserves physical health but also contributes to emotional comfort, as many elderly women fear the loss of dignity due to hygiene challenges.

Bathing should be done regularly, but it's also important to strike a balance between keeping them clean and respecting their privacy. Some elderly people may feel uncomfortable with someone else assisting them with such personal tasks. You can offer to use a handheld showerhead or provide towels for them to cover up during bathing to preserve their modesty.

Skin Care and Hydration

As people age, their skin becomes more fragile and prone to dryness or irritation. A good skincare routine can prevent issues like cracking or infections. Make sure to apply moisturizing lotion to keep their skin hydrated and healthy, especially after bathing.

Encourage them to drink water throughout the day, as dehydration can cause a range of health problems, from dry skin to more serious issues like confusion or urinary tract infections. It can be easy for seniors to forget to drink water, so offer fluids regularly and make it a part of their daily routine.

Dressing and Grooming

Helping your elderly loved one get dressed or groomed each day can be a chance for them to feel more independent and dignified. Whenever possible, encourage them to take part in these tasks. If they struggle with buttons or zippers, opt for clothing that is easier to put on, like loose-fitting pants with elastic waistbands or tops with Velcro closures.

Regular grooming, such as brushing their hair or trimming their nails, also contributes to their self-esteem. You can turn this into a bonding moment—perhaps by setting up a "salon day" where you do their hair or nails, which can make them feel pampered and special.

Practical Tips for Physical Care:

- Establish a consistent daily routine that includes hygiene, mobility, and hydration.

- Change their position regularly to prevent bed sores and encourage gentle movement whenever possible.

- Maintain proper hygiene, especially for women, to prevent infections, and respect their modesty.

- Moisturize their skin and encourage hydration throughout the day.

- Assist with dressing and grooming in a way that promotes independence and dignity.

Providing physical care can be one of the more demanding aspects of caregiving, but it's also one of the most important. By creating a daily routine that prioritizes comfort, hygiene, and mobility, you'll not only ensure their health but also help preserve their dignity and self-esteem.

Caring for a loved one with dementia or Alzheimer's is a unique challenge, requiring patience, empathy, and adaptability. As memory fades and confusion sets in, both the caregiver and the person in care face emotional and practical obstacles that can be overwhelming. In this chapter, we'll explore the specific challenges of dementia care, how to manage difficult behaviors, and ways to create a calm, safe environment for those living with these conditions.

The Challenges of Dementia Care

Dementia, especially Alzheimer's disease, impacts both memory and behavior. Over time, those affected may forget familiar faces, places, and even how to perform basic daily tasks. This can create deep frustration for the person with dementia and emotional strain for their caregivers, who must learn to navigate these changes while preserving the dignity of their loved ones.

The progression of the disease can lead to repeated questions, wandering, agitation, and even aggressive behavior. Caregivers often feel a sense of loss, as the person they once knew seems to slip away gradually. It's common to experience feelings of sadness, frustration, and even burnout.

Understanding that these behaviors are symptoms of the illness and not intentional is crucial to providing compassionate care. The key is finding ways to support your loved one while managing the emotional and physical toll dementia care can take on caregivers.

Tips for Managing Difficult Behaviors:

Dealing with difficult behaviors in dementia patients can be one of the hardest aspects of caregiving. However, there are strategies to ease the burden and reduce stress for both the caregiver and the patient:

1. Remain Calm and Patient: Dementia can make communication challenging. Repeating the same questions or expressing confusion isn't done to frustrate you—it's part of their condition. Answer calmly and simply, even if it's for the hundredth time. Losing patience can escalate their anxiety.

2. Redirect, Don't Argue: It's tempting to correct or argue when a person with dementia becomes confused or insists on something untrue. However, it's often more effective to gently redirect the conversation. If your loved one insists they need to leave for work, for example, you could redirect by saying, "Let's have a cup of tea first," instead of arguing that they are retired.

3. Establish a Routine: People with dementia thrive on routine. Predictable daily activities can help reduce confusion and anxiety. Simple routines, like waking up at the same time or eating meals at consistent times, provide a sense of structure.

4. Use Visual Cues: Dementia can cause people to lose track of where they are or what they're supposed to do next. Using visual aids like clocks, labeled drawers, and calendars can help them feel more grounded and reduce confusion.

5. Limit Stimulation: Agitation can be triggered by loud noises, too many visitors, or unfamiliar environments. When they become upset, try reducing stimuli by turning off the TV, dimming the lights, or moving to a quieter space. A peaceful, calm environment can help them feel safe and less overwhelmed.

Creating a Safe Environment

Safety is a critical concern when caring for someone with dementia. Their memory loss and confusion can lead to wandering, accidents, and other dangerous situations. Here are some steps to help ensure their safety:

1. Secure the Home: Dementia patients may wander off, which can be extremely dangerous. Install locks on doors and windows, or use monitoring devices to keep track of your loved one's movements. You may also want to alert neighbors so they can help watch out for them.

2. Reduce Fall Risks: Dementia can affect balance and coordination. Remove tripping hazards like loose rugs, electrical cords, or clutter from walking paths. Installing grab bars in the bathroom and using non-slip mats in the shower can also help prevent accidents.

3. Simplify the Environment: As dementia progresses, too much visual clutter can lead to confusion. Keep their living space simple, organized, and free from unnecessary objects. Clearly labeled drawers and cupboards can help them find things without frustration.

4. Use Safety Devices: Consider adding safety devices like stove guards to prevent accidental fires or automatic shut-off devices for appliances. Ensure medications are locked away, as dementia patients may forget their dosage or take the wrong pills.

5. Monitor for Wandering: Wandering is common in dementia patients, especially in the later stages. If possible, create a safe, enclosed outdoor space where they can move freely without getting lost. If wandering remains an issue, you might need to explore GPS trackers or in-home monitoring systems for added peace of mind.

Coping with the Emotional Toll

Caring for a loved one with dementia can be emotionally draining, especially when behaviors become difficult or the disease progresses rapidly. Caregivers need to acknowledge their own needs and seek support:

Take Breaks: Caring for someone with dementia is exhausting. Make sure to take regular breaks to recharge, even if it means arranging respite care for a day or two.

Seek Support Groups: Talking with other caregivers who are going through the same experience can provide emotional relief and practical tips. Many communities offer support groups for dementia caregivers.

Practice Self-Compassion: Feelings of guilt, frustration, or helplessness are common in dementia care. It's important to remember that you're doing the best you can. Be kind to yourself and seek help when needed.

Final Thoughts

Caring for someone with dementia or Alzheimer's is an intense and challenging journey, but it's also an opportunity to show deep compassion and love. By understanding the condition, managing difficult behaviors with patience, and creating a safe and calm environment, you can help your loved one live as comfortably as possible. Remember to also take care of yourself along the way—seeking support is key to avoiding burnout and providing the best care possible.

Proper nutrition and hydration play a pivotal role in maintaining an elderly person's health. However, as people age, their dietary needs change, and it can be a challenge to ensure they are eating balanced meals that support their overall well-being. Factors like reduced appetite, dental issues, or medical conditions can make it difficult for seniors to get the nutrients they need. As their caregiver, you play an important role in helping them maintain a healthy diet.

Understanding Their Nutritional Needs

Elderly individuals often require fewer calories than younger adults due to a slower metabolism and reduced physical activity. However, they still need plenty of vitamins, minerals, and protein to keep their bodies strong. Make sure their diet is rich in fruits, vegetables, lean proteins, whole grains, and healthy fats.

Protein, in particular, is crucial for preventing muscle loss, which can lead to frailty and falls. Incorporate protein sources like chicken, fish, eggs, and beans into their meals. If they struggle with chewing or swallowing, you can use softer foods like scrambled eggs, yogurt, or smoothies to meet their nutritional needs.

Calcium and vitamin D are also important for bone health, as aging bones become more prone to fractures. Include dairy products like milk and cheese or fortified alternatives to ensure they get enough calcium. Supplements might also be necessary, depending on their diet.

Dealing with Reduced Appetite

One of the most common issues in elderly care is reduced appetite. Your loved one might not feel hungry as often, or they may find it difficult to enjoy food the way they used to. There are several reasons for this, including medications, dental problems, or changes in taste and smell.

To encourage eating, try to make meals as appealing as possible. Serve smaller, nutrient-dense meals more frequently rather than three large meals a day. You can also offer snacks like nuts, cheese, or fruit throughout the day to help them get the calories and nutrients they need. Meals that are colorful and visually appealing may also stimulate their appetite.

Make sure the foods you offer are easy to chew and swallow, especially if they have dental issues. Soft foods, like mashed potatoes, oatmeal, or smoothies, can be both nutritious and easier for them to eat. Pay attention to any signs of difficulty swallowing, such as coughing during meals, and consult with their doctor if needed.

Staying Hydrated

Hydration is just as important as nutrition, but it's often overlooked. As people age, their sense of thirst diminishes, and they may not realize they're becoming dehydrated. Dehydration can lead to serious health problems, including confusion, urinary tract infections, and kidney issues.

Encourage your loved one to drink water regularly throughout the day. If they're resistant to drinking plain water, offer alternatives like herbal teas, diluted fruit juice, or water-rich foods such as watermelon, cucumbers, and soups. Make sure fluids are readily accessible, especially if they have limited mobility. Placing water bottles or cups within reach can serve as a reminder to drink.

Special Dietary Considerations

If your loved one has specific health conditions, such as diabetes, high blood pressure, or heart disease, their diet may need to be adjusted accordingly. Work with a healthcare professional to develop a meal plan that supports their medical needs. For instance, if they have diabetes, it's important to control carbohydrate intake and monitor blood sugar levels. For those with high blood pressure, reducing salt intake can help manage the condition.

In some cases, supplements may be necessary to meet their nutritional needs. Speak with their doctor about vitamins or supplements like vitamin D, calcium, or omega-3 fatty acids, especially if they're not getting enough from food.

Maintaining a Sense of Independence

Whenever possible, involve your loved one in their meal planning and preparation. Even if they can't cook, asking them about their favorite foods or letting them help with simple tasks like stirring a pot or setting the table can give them a sense of control and independence. This also makes mealtime a more enjoyable and social experience, rather than a chore.

Practical Tips for Nutrition and Hydration:

- Provide nutrient-dense meals with plenty of protein, fruits, vegetables, and whole grains.

- Offer smaller, frequent meals if they struggle with appetite, and use soft foods if chewing is an issue.

- Keep them hydrated by offering water and hydrating foods throughout the day.

- Adjust their diet according to any health conditions, with guidance from a healthcare professional.

- Involve them in meal planning or preparation to promote a sense of independence.

Nutrition and hydration are vital to your loved one's well-being, and as their caregiver, your attention to these details will greatly impact their quality of life.

As our loved ones age, their dietary needs change, and ensuring they get proper nutrition can be a challenge. Physical changes, medical conditions, and medications can all impact appetite, digestion, and nutrient absorption. In this chapter, we'll focus on the importance of nutrition and meal planning for the elderly, offering practical tips to keep your loved one well-nourished while considering their preferences, health needs, and ability to prepare food.

The Importance of Nutrition in Elder Care

Good nutrition is essential at any stage of life, but for older adults, it becomes even more critical. Eating the right foods can help manage chronic conditions such as diabetes, heart disease, and high blood pressure, while also supporting their immune system and overall well-being. Proper nutrition helps maintain strength, bone health, cognitive function, and energy levels, reducing the risk of illness and falls.

However, many elderly people experience reduced appetite or difficulty preparing meals due to physical limitations, which can lead to poor nutrition or even malnutrition. You may notice that your loved one is eating less or favoring processed or easy-to-prepare meals that lack the necessary vitamins and minerals. This is where thoughtful meal planning can make a significant difference.

Tailoring Meals to Their Needs

When planning meals, it's important to consider your loved one's unique dietary needs, preferences, and any medical conditions they may have. Consulting with a doctor or nutritionist can provide valuable guidance on what types of foods are best for them. For example, someone with diabetes may need to monitor their carbohydrate intake, while a person with high blood pressure should limit their salt intake.

Incorporating nutrient-dense foods into their diet is key. Focus on whole foods such as lean proteins (chicken, fish, beans), whole grains (oats, brown rice, quinoa), and fresh fruits and vegetables. These provide essential vitamins, minerals, and fiber while being easier to digest. For those with dental issues, soft-cooked vegetables, stews, and smoothies can be a great way to get the necessary nutrients without causing discomfort.

Overcoming Appetite Loss

Many elderly people experience a decrease in appetite, which can result in weight loss and nutritional deficiencies. There are several reasons for this, including changes in taste, smell, or the side effects of medication. Eating can also become less enjoyable if they have difficulty chewing or swallowing.

To encourage your loved one to eat more, try offering smaller, more frequent meals throughout the day rather than sticking to three large meals. Finger foods, snacks like yogurt, cheese, or fruit, and nutrient-rich soups can help them maintain their caloric intake without overwhelming them. Experiment with herbs and spices to enhance the flavor of foods if their taste buds have changed, and make mealtimes as pleasant and stress-free as possible.

Hydration is Key

Staying hydrated is just as important as getting the right nutrition, yet many elderly people don't drink enough water. Dehydration can cause confusion, urinary tract infections, and even hospitalizations. Encourage your loved one to drink fluids throughout the day, and offer a variety of hydrating options like water, herbal teas, broths, or water-rich foods like fruits and vegetables.

If your loved one struggles with drinking plain water, try infusing it with slices of lemon, cucumber, or berries for added flavor. Be mindful of beverages with too much caffeine or sugar, as these can lead to dehydration or spikes in blood sugar.

Meal Preparation and Accessibility

As your loved one ages, preparing meals may become more difficult due to physical limitations or cognitive decline. If they struggle with meal preparation, consider simplifying the process by preparing meals in advance or making larger batches that can be frozen and reheated later. This ensures that they have nutritious meals ready to go when they are hungry, without the effort of cooking from scratch.

You can also make their kitchen more accessible by organizing it in a way that allows them to reach important items easily. Keep their favorite snacks and ingredients within arm's reach, and use adaptive kitchen tools like easy-grip utensils or electric can openers to reduce the strain of meal preparation.

If meal preparation is no longer possible for them, look into meal delivery services or community programs which offer nutritious meals specifically tailored for seniors. These options ensure your loved one continues to receive balanced, delicious meals even if they can no longer cook for themselves.

Special Considerations: Memory Loss and Dementia

For those with memory loss or dementia, meal times can be especially challenging. They may forget to eat, lose interest in food, or become confused about when and what to eat. Establishing a regular meal schedule can help, and using visual cues—such as setting the table at the same time each day—can signal that it's time to eat.

Offer simple, familiar foods that they've always enjoyed, and avoid overwhelming them with too many choices. If they have difficulty using utensils, finger foods like sandwiches, cut-up vegetables, or fruit slices may make eating easier. Be patient, and give them plenty of time to finish their meal without feeling rushed.

Involving Them in Meal Decisions

Whenever possible, involve your loved one in meal planning and preparation. This gives them a sense of control over their diet and helps them stay engaged with food. Ask for their input on what they would like to eat, offer them choices, and involve them in simple tasks like stirring ingredients or setting the table.

By allowing them to make decisions about their meals, you help them maintain their independence and ensure they are eating foods they enjoy. Even small acts of participation can make a big difference in how they feel about mealtime.

Practical Tips for Managing Nutrition:

- Focus on nutrient-dense foods, including lean proteins, whole grains, and fresh fruits and vegetables.

- Offer smaller, more frequent meals if they have a reduced appetite.

- Encourage hydration with water, herbal teas, and water-rich foods.

- Simplify meal preparation with pre-prepared meals or meal delivery services.

- Involve them in meal planning to give them a sense of control and independence.

- Establish regular meal routines, especially for those with memory loss.

Proper nutrition is fundamental to maintaining your loved one's health, energy, and overall quality of life. By taking a thoughtful approach to meal planning and preparation, you can ensure that they receive the nourishment they need, even as their tastes and abilities change with age.

One of the most critical aspects of elder care is managing medications. As people age, they often need a variety of medications for chronic health conditions, from high blood pressure to diabetes or arthritis. It can be overwhelming to keep track of them all, especially if your loved one is on multiple medications with different dosages and schedules. Proper management is essential not only for their health but also to avoid dangerous mistakes.

Creating a Medication Schedule

The first step in managing medications is to create a schedule that clearly outlines what needs to be taken and when. Use a simple chart or a pill organizer that breaks down doses by day and time. Many caregivers find that using a pill organizer with compartments for morning, afternoon, and evening doses helps minimize confusion.

If your elderly loved one has memory problems, they might forget whether they've taken their medication. A clear, visible chart or digital reminder system can help keep both of you on track. For those who use smartphones or tablets, setting alarms for medication times can also be helpful.

Understanding the Medications

It's important to understand each medication's purpose, dosage, and potential side effects. Speak with their doctor or pharmacist to clarify why each drug is necessary and how it interacts with others. Some medications may have side effects like dizziness or drowsiness, which could increase the risk of falls, while others might need to be taken with food to avoid stomach upset. Understanding these details ensures that you're not only giving medications correctly but also taking steps to minimize side effects.

Keep a list of all current medications, including over-the-counter drugs, vitamins, and supplements, and update it whenever there's a change. This list should be easily accessible and shared with doctors or other caregivers to avoid any confusion during medical visits.

Avoiding Dangerous Interactions

Elderly individuals are at higher risk of adverse drug interactions due to the number of medications they often take. Make sure their doctor is aware of all medications and supplements they are taking, as some combinations can cause harmful side effects. For example, certain blood pressure medications may interact poorly with over-the-counter cold medicines or supplements like St. John's Wort can interfere with prescription drugs.

Before starting any new medication or supplement, consult with a healthcare professional to ensure it won't negatively affect their existing regimen. It's also helpful to use a single pharmacy for all prescriptions, as the pharmacist will have a complete record of their medications and can alert you to any potential issues.

Involving Them in the Process

Even if your loved one has cognitive or physical limitations, it's important to involve them in their medication routine as much as possible. If they are able, encourage them to participate in sorting their pills or tracking doses. This fosters a sense of control and can help reduce any feelings of helplessness that often come with aging.

For those dealing with memory loss, you may need to be more hands-on in managing their medication schedule, but always explain what you're doing and why. For example, say, "It's time for your blood pressure medication. This helps keep your heart healthy." Keeping them informed, even if they forget quickly, shows respect for their autonomy

Keeping Medications Secure

Some elderly individuals may become confused or forgetful, which can lead to taking too much or too little of their medication. In these cases, it's vital to store medications in a safe place, away from where they might accidentally access them. Consider locking medications away if there's a risk they might try to take them on their own and get confused about dosages.

If your loved one has difficulty swallowing pills, ask their doctor or pharmacist if the medication can be crushed, taken in liquid form, or if there are alternative options available. Always consult a healthcare professional before altering the form of any medication.

Practical Tips for Medication Management:

- Create a visible medication schedule or use a pill organizer to stay on track.

- Keep an up-to-date list of all medications, including supplements, and share it with healthcare providers.

- Be aware of potential interactions and side effects by consulting with a doctor or pharmacist.

- Involve your loved one in the medication process whenever possible to promote autonomy.

- Store medications securely and consult professionals if your loved one has trouble taking them.

Medication management is essential to keeping your elderly loved one healthy and safe. By staying organized, informed, and vigilant about potential interactions, you can ensure that their medications work effectively and without complications.

As important as physical health is for the elderly, their mental and emotional well-being is just as critical. Aging can bring about challenges like memory loss, loneliness, and depression, which affect their overall quality of life. Keeping their minds stimulated and fostering emotional connections can greatly improve their outlook and health. In this chapter, we'll explore strategies for maintaining their cognitive function and emotional balance.

Combating Loneliness and Isolation

One of the greatest challenges elderly individuals face is loneliness. Many find themselves living apart from their families, losing friends, or becoming isolated due to mobility issues. This isolation can lead to feelings of sadness and depression, which may, in turn, affect their physical health.

To prevent this, make a concerted effort to include your loved one in family activities, even if they can no longer participate as fully as they once did. A simple phone call or video chat can brighten their day. Visits, even short ones, are incredibly valuable. During these visits, encourage conversations about their past, their interests, and what brings them joy. This can help them feel more connected and valued.

Engaging with their local community can also be a powerful way to combat loneliness. Senior centers, book clubs, or religious gatherings can provide a space for socialization and new friendships. If they can't leave the house often, consider virtual options that allow them to engage with others from the comfort of home.

Stimulating Their Minds

Keeping the mind active is essential for cognitive health. Studies have shown that engaging in mentally stimulating activities can slow down memory loss and even delay the onset of dementia. Encourage your loved one to engage in activities they enjoy that challenge their brain. Puzzles, card games, and word games are all great options for exercising mental sharpness.

Reading, in particular, can be a wonderful way to keep their minds engaged. If their eyesight has weakened, audiobooks or having someone read to them can still allow them to enjoy books. Choose material that they love—whether it's their favorite mystery novels, their bible, or stories from their youth. The familiarity can spark joy and bring back fond memories.

In addition to traditional activities, consider introducing new hobbies that stimulate their brain in different ways. Knitting, painting, or even learning basic technology skills can challenge their cognitive abilities while giving them a sense of accomplishment.

Dealing with Memory Loss

Memory loss can be one of the most difficult changes to navigate as a caregiver. If your loved one is struggling with forgetfulness or a more serious form of cognitive decline, like Alzheimer's or dementia, it requires extra patience and understanding.

When interacting with someone experiencing memory loss, try to keep communication simple and clear. Avoid overwhelming them with too many details at once. Gentle reminders, rather than corrections, can help maintain their dignity. For example, instead of saying, "You already asked that," try, "Let me tell you about it again."

It's also helpful to establish a routine. Having a predictable schedule can reduce confusion and anxiety for your loved one. Use visual aids, like calendars or written reminders, to help them remember daily tasks or upcoming appointments. As memory loss progresses, it's important to find a balance between supporting their independence and providing necessary care.

Staying Emotionally Connected

As a caregiver, you're not just providing physical support—you're also a source of emotional connection. Being present, listening, and validating your loved one's feelings can make a huge difference in their emotional well-being. Take time to sit and talk with them, even if the conversation is brief. These moments of connection are vital for their mental health and remind them that they are loved and valued.

At the same time, it's important to acknowledge that caring for someone with emotional or cognitive challenges can be taxing. Be sure to look after your emotional well-being as well. Don't hesitate to ask for help from other family members or seek support from caregiving groups when you need it.

Providing Entertainment

Keeping your loved one entertained is a key component of their emotional well-being. Beyond mental stimulation, they need activities that make them feel joy and fulfillment. If they enjoy music, playing their favorite songs or encouraging them to sing along can lift their spirits. Watching movies or television shows they love can also be a source of comfort.

You can also keep them entertained by involving them in activities that give them a sense of purpose. Tasks like helping fold laundry, organizing photo albums, or even planning a family meal together can be fulfilling. Even though they might not be able to do everything on their own, the sense of contribution can brighten their mood and make them feel useful.

Practical Tips for Mental and Emotional Well-being:

- Schedule regular family visits or calls to combat loneliness and encourage community engagement.

- Keep their minds stimulated with games, puzzles, reading, and new hobbies.

- Use gentle reminders and clear communication for those with memory loss.

- Establish a routine and use visual aids to reduce confusion.

- Offer entertainment that brings them joy, like music, movies, or helping with simple tasks.

Mental and emotional health are crucial to your loved one's overall well-being. As their caregiver, you play a key role in providing them with the social interaction, mental stimulation, and emotional connection they need to thrive.

One of the most challenging aspects of elder care is finding the right balance between respecting your loved one's independence and ensuring their safety. Many elderly people desire to remain in their own homes and continue managing their affairs, but as health and mobility decline, this can become increasingly difficult. In this chapter, we'll explore how to handle these difficult conversations and help your loved one feel secure and respected, even when it's time to make tough decisions.

The Emotional Aspect of Losing Independence

Losing the ability to live independently can be an emotionally painful experience for your loved one. They may feel frustrated, scared, or even angry at the prospect of needing help, especially if they have always been self-reliant. Understanding this emotional journey can help you approach the situation with empathy and compassion.

It's crucial to acknowledge that for many elderly people, their home is not just a place but a symbol of their freedom and identity. Moving out or accepting assistance may feel like they are losing control of their life, and this can stir up feelings of fear, grief, or inadequacy.

Gentle and Open Communication

When discussing matters of safety and care with your loved one, approach the conversation with patience and understanding. Start by expressing your concern for their well-being, emphasizing that your main goal is to support them, not to take away their independence.

For example, if your loved one wants to continue living on their own, but you have concerns about their safety, gently explain that you are not trying to take away their freedom. Instead, reassure them that your intentions are to find solutions that will allow them to live as independently as possible while still staying safe. This can help ease their anxieties and open the door to more productive conversations.

Assessing Safety and Making Practical Adjustments

If your loved one's home is becoming less safe for them to navigate, it's worth looking into practical adjustments that can make it easier for them to stay there. Consider installing safety features such as grab bars in the bathroom, non-slip mats, and better lighting throughout the home. Rearranging furniture to minimize tripping hazards or moving essential items to lower, more accessible shelves can also make a big difference.

Additionally, if mobility is a concern, hiring a part-time caregiver or organizing family support can help ensure that they receive the assistance they need while still maintaining as much independence as possible.

When It's Time for a Transition

In some cases, it may no longer be practical for your loved one to live alone, and the time may come to discuss alternative living arrangements, such as moving in with family or considering an assisted living facility. These discussions are often the most difficult, as they can feel like a loss of autonomy to the elderly person.

If you've reached this stage, approach the topic gently, and give your loved one plenty of time to adjust to the idea. Discuss the benefits of the new arrangement, such as increased safety, social opportunities, and access to care. Frame the conversation around their comfort and quality of life rather than focusing on their limitations.

Wherever possible, involve them in the decision-making process. Visit assisted living facilities together or discuss potential modifications to your home to accommodate their needs. The more control they feel they have over the situation, the more likely they are to accept the change with grace.

Supporting Them Through the Transition

Moving or accepting help can be an emotionally taxing experience for your loved one, so offering ongoing support is essential. Help them adjust to their new environment, whether it's a new home or accepting more care within their current residence. Stay connected with them, visit regularly, and ensure they still have a say in decisions about their care and lifestyle.

Remind them that needing assistance is not a failure, but a natural part of aging. Aging comes with many transitions, and each one can be managed with dignity and love. Your support will go a long way in making this new chapter of their life as positive and fulfilling as possible.

Encouraging Independence in New Ways

Even if your loved one is no longer able to live entirely on their own, there are still plenty of ways to foster independence in their daily life. Encourage them to participate in activities that they enjoy, help them stay connected with friends and family, and continue to give them autonomy over decisions that matter to them, such as meal preferences or how they spend their leisure time.

By respecting their wishes and empowering them in whatever ways possible, you can help them maintain their sense of identity and purpose even as their living situation changes.

Practical Tips for Balancing Independence and Safety:

- Acknowledge the emotional difficulty of losing independence and approach conversations with empathy.

- Reassure them that your goal is to support them, not take away their freedom.

- Consider practical safety adjustments in their home to allow them to live independently longer.

- Involve them in decisions about care and living arrangements whenever possible.

- Offer emotional and practical support through any transitions, helping them adjust with dignity.

- Foster independence in new ways, ensuring they still have a voice in their care.

Elder care introduces a new chapter in family dynamics, one where roles evolve and relationships are tested. As family members adjust to caregiving responsibilities, it's common for emotional strain and conflict to surface. However, with patience, open communication, and clear planning, these challenges can be navigated successfully. In this chapter, we'll dive into how caregiving affects family dynamics, how to handle conflicts, and strategies for managing emotions that come with this difficult but meaningful responsibility.

Understanding the Family Dynamics of Caregiving

When a family member takes on the role of primary caregiver for an elderly relative, the entire family system can be affected. Long-standing family roles may shift, and new tensions can arise. Adult children may find themselves in an unfamiliar position, reversing the caretaker dynamic they had with their parent. The emotional weight of this role reversal can be overwhelming, particularly when juggling work, children, and other commitments.

Siblings often have varying opinions on what is best for their aging parent, and disagreements can occur. One sibling might feel the burden of being the primary caregiver, while another sibling might not be as involved, creating friction. Without proper communication, feelings of resentment can deepen, straining the family bond.

Navigating Conflicts Between Siblings and Parents

Sibling rivalry often resurfaces in elder care, especially when the caregiving responsibilities are not equally shared. One sibling may take on most of the work, which can lead to feelings of frustration if they feel unsupported by other family members. On the other hand, a sibling who is less involved might feel left out of decision-making processes, causing tension.

Open and honest communication is essential to prevent misunderstandings from escalating. Families should have regular conversations about caregiving duties and ensure that everyone's opinion is valued. If possible, consider dividing responsibilities according to each sibling's strengths. One might handle finances, while another takes on the medical side, and others assist with social or emotional support. Having a clear plan can alleviate feelings of being overwhelmed and reduce conflict.

It's also important to include the elderly parent in these conversations as much as possible. Even if they need more help than before, allowing them a voice in their own care decisions can foster mutual respect and reduce the strain of decision-making on the caregiver.

Tips for Dividing Caregiving Responsibilities

Caregiving is a team effort, and it's important to divide responsibilities in a way that feels fair to everyone involved. Here are some tips to make this process smoother:

1. Assess Everyone's Availability: It's important to acknowledge that everyone has different time commitments. Some family members may have demanding jobs or live far away, while others might be more available. Be realistic about what each person can contribute.

2. Leverage Strengths: Think about who is best suited for certain tasks. If one sibling is good with finances, they might manage the budget and insurance paperwork. Another who lives nearby might focus on errands, doctor's appointments, and visits. Sharing the load based on strengths helps ensure tasks are done

well without burning out any one person.

3. Schedule Regular Check-Ins: Keep lines of communication open by having family meetings or calls to discuss how the care plan is working and whether any adjustments need to be made. This helps prevent small grievances from becoming major sources of tension.

4. Don't Be Afraid to Ask for Help: If caregiving becomes too overwhelming, consider professional support like in-home care, respite care, or adult day services. Bringing in outside help can relieve some of the pressure on family members, especially if no one has the time or skills to meet all the needs.

Managing Resentment, Guilt, and Frustration

Feelings of resentment, guilt, and frustration are common in caregiving, especially when family members feel overburdened or unsupported. It's important to recognize these emotions and address them early to prevent them from festering and damaging relationships.

Resentment can stem from feeling like one person is shouldering the bulk of the caregiving duties. To alleviate this, be honest about your limits and ask for help when needed. Discuss responsibilities with your siblings or other family members and ensure that caregiving is as balanced as possible.

Guilt is often felt when caregivers feel like they're not doing enough or are stretched too thin between caregiving and other obligations. It's important to remember that no one can do everything perfectly. Seek professional support when necessary, and remind yourself that doing your best is enough.

Frustration often arises when caregiving becomes physically or emotionally exhausting, especially if the care recipient has memory loss or other cognitive challenges. Patience is key, but so is taking time for self-care. Make sure you're setting aside moments to recharge, whether that's through taking a walk, spending time with friends, or simply resting.

Strengthening Family Bonds Through Caregiving
While caregiving can strain family relationships, it can also strengthen them. By working together, family members can reconnect and create new, meaningful memories with their elderly loved one. Sharing stories, reminiscing, and celebrating small victories in caregiving can bring family members closer together and help ease the stress of this responsibility.

Caregiving is a journey which requires empathy, patience, and ongoing support from all family members. By maintaining open lines of communication and supporting each other emotionally and practically, families can weather the challenges of elder care with grace and compassion.

Final Thoughts

Family roles shift when elder care becomes necessary, and it's natural for emotions to run high. By maintaining healthy communication, dividing responsibilities, and addressing negative feelings like resentment or guilt, you can manage the emotional and practical aspects of caregiving. Ultimately, navigating this journey together can lead to stronger family relationships and a more fulfilling caregiving experience.

Caring for an elderly loved one is a noble and compassionate act, but it can also be physically, emotionally, and mentally draining. Without adequate self-care, the pressures of caregiving can quickly lead to burnout, affecting your ability to care for others and yourself. In this chapter, we'll focus on why self-care is essential for caregivers, practical ways to manage stress and prevent burnout, and how to balance your life and responsibilities effectively.

Preventing Caregiver Burnout

Caregiver burnout is a state of physical, emotional, and mental exhaustion that occurs when the demands of caregiving become overwhelming. It's easy to neglect your own needs when you're constantly caring for someone else, but doing so can have serious consequences for your health and well-being.

Burnout doesn't happen overnight—it creeps in slowly as stress accumulates. Common signs include feeling constantly tired, becoming irritable or short-tempered, losing interest in activities you once enjoyed, and feeling helpless or hopeless. If left unchecked, burnout can lead to depression, anxiety, and even physical illness.

How to recognize burnout:

- Emotional Exhaustion: Feeling drained and unable to cope with daily tasks.

- Detachment: Becoming distant from the person you are caring for or feeling numb.

- Physical Symptoms: Frequent headaches, stomach problems, or muscle pain due to stress.

- Feeling Trapped: Feeling like there's no way out or that caregiving is taking over your life.

It's important to acknowledge these signs early and take action before burnout worsens. Remember, caring for yourself isn't a luxury—it's a necessity. When you're at your best, you can provide better care for your loved one.

Practical Ways to Care for Yourself

Self-care isn't about taking lavish vacations or indulging in spa days (though those things are great when you can manage them). It's about finding small, meaningful ways to recharge, relieve stress, and maintain balance in your life. Here are some practical tips for incorporating self-care into your routine:

1. Schedule Breaks: Taking short breaks throughout the day can help reset your mind and body. Even five minutes of quiet time can make a difference. Step outside for fresh air, enjoy a cup of tea or practice deep breathing exercises.

2. Delegate Tasks: Don't be afraid to ask for help. Family members, friends, or even professional caregivers can share some of the load. If others are willing to pitch in, let them. It's okay to accept help, whether it's with grocery shopping, cleaning, or providing care for a few hours.

3. Stay Connected: Social isolation is a common problem for caregivers. Make an effort to stay connected with friends and family, even if it's just through a phone call or text message. Talking to someone who understands your situation can provide emotional relief and reduce feelings of loneliness.

4. Exercise Regularly: Physical activity is a great way to relieve stress and boost your mood. You don't have to spend hours at the gym—even a 20-minute walk around your neighborhood can help clear your mind and improve your physical health.

5. Practice Mindfulness or Meditation: Mindfulness and meditation can help you stay present and reduce anxiety. Even a few minutes of focused breathing or sitting in quiet reflection can improve your mental clarity and help you manage stressful situations.

6. Set Realistic Expectations: Caregiving can be overwhelming, and it's important to acknowledge that you can't do everything perfectly. Set realistic goals for yourself and your loved one's care. It's okay to lower expectations when needed and accept that some days will be harder than others.

7. Sleep and Nutrition: Proper sleep and nutrition are the foundation of self-care. Make sure you're getting enough rest, eating balanced meals, and staying hydrated. If you're struggling with sleep, try establishing a bedtime routine or using relaxation techniques to wind down at the end of the day.

Finding Support

No caregiver should go through the process alone. Support is essential, both in practical and emotional terms. There are several ways to build a support network that can help you manage the stresses of caregiving:

Support Groups: Joining a caregiver support group, whether in person or online, can provide a sense of community and shared understanding. You can exchange tips, offer advice, and find comfort in knowing you're not alone in your struggles.

Respite Care: Respite care provides short-term relief for caregivers by giving them a break while a professional caregiver takes over for a few hours or days. It's an excellent way to recharge without feeling guilty about stepping away.

Counseling: If you're struggling with the emotional toll of caregiving, talking to a therapist can help. They can provide tools for managing stress, navigating family dynamics, and addressing feelings of guilt or resentment.

Friends and Family: Don't hesitate to lean on your friends and family for emotional support. Even if they can't help with caregiving, talking about your feelings and frustrations can lighten your emotional burden.

Balancing Life and Responsibilities

Balancing caregiving with your personal life, job, or other responsibilities can feel like an impossible task. However, finding a balance is key to preventing burnout and maintaining a sense of control over your life.

1. Create a Routine: Establishing a daily routine for both you and your loved one can create structure and reduce stress. When tasks are scheduled, it's easier to prioritize and manage time.

2. Set Boundaries: It's important to set boundaries with both your loved one and other family members. Know when to say no, and make sure you're not taking on more than you can handle. Healthy boundaries ensure that your needs aren't overlooked.

3. Prioritize Tasks: Some days, you may not be able to accomplish everything. Focus on the most important tasks first, and give yourself permission to let less urgent things slide. Accept that you can't do it all and that's okay.

4. Carve Out "Me Time": Even if it's just 15 minutes a day, find time to do something you enjoy—whether it's reading a book, taking a

walk, or listening to music. These small breaks can help you feel more balanced and in control.

Final Thoughts

Self-care isn't selfish—it's essential. As a caregiver, you have the responsibility not only to care for your loved one but also to care for yourself. By managing stress, seeking support, and finding balance, you can provide better care for your loved one while maintaining your own well-being. Remember, it's okay to ask for help and take time for yourself. In the long run, it will make you a stronger, more resilient caregiver.

CONCLUSION

Caring for an elderly loved one requires a delicate balance of compassion, patience, and practicality. The journey is often filled with both emotional and physical demands, as you navigate the complexities of ensuring their safety, maintaining their independence, and adapting to their changing needs. These challenges may seem overwhelming at times, but they also present opportunities for growth, connection, and deeper understanding.

The heart of elder care lies in empathy. By keeping the lines of communication open and approaching each situation with grace, it's possible to not only meet the practical needs of our elderly loved ones but also honor their dignity and wishes. Every act of care, no matter how small, is a testament to love and respect for the lives they've lived and the journeys they continue to take.

I want to express my deepest gratitude to you, the reader, for joining me on this meaningful path. The experience of elder care is not a one-size-fits-all, and I hope the insights shared in these chapters have resonated with you, offering both guidance and comfort. Whether you are just beginning or are well along the caregiving road, may these reflections provide encouragement, inspiration, and practical tips to help you navigate the way forward.

Remember that in caring for others, you are also taking part in a shared human experience—one of kindness, resilience, and commitment. Each day brings its own set of challenges, but with patience, compassion, and wisdom, you will find your way through.

Thank you for your dedication to this vital and heartfelt work.

BOOKS BY THIS AUTHOR

Finding My Way Around Midlife

State Of The Union: Working At It